How to Ride Your Own Personal Stress Wave - and Thrive!

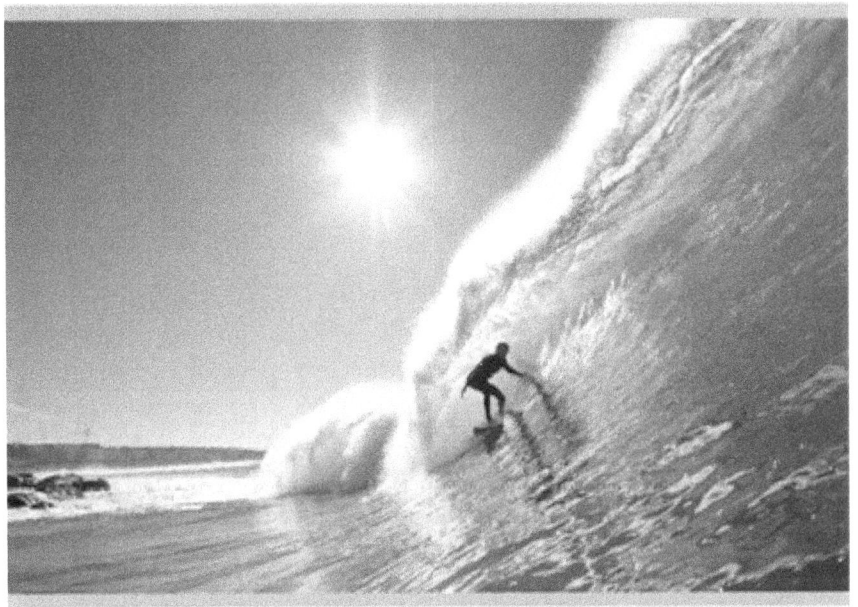

DR. ROY VARTABEDIAN
DEBI SILBER, MS, RD

First Edition
Copyright © August 2017
by Dr. Roy E. Vartabedian
and Debi Silber, MS, RD, WHC

ISBN: 978-1548668464

Designs for Wellness Press
P.O. Box 1144
Prosper, TX 75078-1144
760-458-4993

The information in this book reflects the authors' experience and current research. It is not intended to be used to replace or supersede individualized medical or professional advice. Before starting any health and wellness program, you should consult a physician or other appropriate health professional to supervise your overall program.

Printed in the United States of America

Visit Dr. Vartabedian's website: www.Nutripoints.com

Visit Debi Silber's website: www.TheMojoCoach.com

How to Ride Your Own Personal Stress Wave and Thrive!

About the Authors

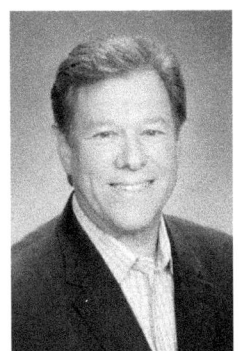

DR. ROY VARTABEDIAN is a specialist in Chronic Disease Prevention and holds a Doctor of Public Health degree from Loma Linda University, and Master of Public Health degrees in Health Education and Nutrition.

He is founder and President of Vartabedian and Associates Designs for Wellness, and has worked in the field of health promotion and disease prevention internationally for over 30 years, working with patients, managing programs, consulting, and speaking throughout the U.S., Canada, Australia and New Zealand. His landmark publication, *Nutripoints*, a New York Times Best-Seller, has been used in a total of 13 countries in 10 languages worldwide (www.Nutripoints.com).

Dr. Vartabedian worked as Executive Director of Wellness Programs at the world-renowned Cooper Clinic in Dallas, Texas. There he worked with Dr. Kenneth Cooper for 6 years to develop the residential Cooper Wellness Program on the 30-acre Cooper Aerobics Center facility.

Earlier in his career, he taught Preventive Care in the Family Practice Residency at Florida Hospital in Orlando, where he trained Family Practice physicians how to incorporate Patient

Education and Preventive Medicine into their practices, and developed the award-winning Preventive Care Learning Center for patients.

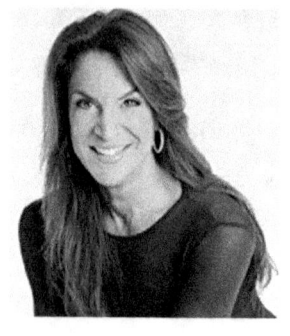 **DEBI SILBER, MS, RD, WHC** The Mojo Coach®, President of Lifestyle Fitness, Inc. and founder of www.TheMojoCoach.com is one of the leading authorities in the fields of health, fitness, wellness and self-improvement. She's a speaker, spokesperson, author of 2 books recommended by Brian Tracy, Marshall Goldsmith, Jack Canfield among others, and is branded The Mojo Coach® because she's personally led hundreds of clients to achieve their ultimate body, mind, image and lifestyle; inspiring them to "get their mojo back" and helping them transform into their personal and professional best.

In addition to receiving honors and awards in the fields of health, business and self-improvement, Debi's contributed to **More Magazine, Working Mother, The National Institute of Health (NIH), Psychology Today, Self, WebMD, Health Magazine, Wellness.com, Yahoo, Wyndham Worldwide, Woman's World** and many more. She's a featured expert on over 15 websites, a popular radio guest, has been featured as a self-improvement expert and successful entrepreneur in 4 books and has a devoted following worldwide. The Mojo Coach® is THE secret behind some of the healthiest, most influential, charismatic, and successful people today who is on a mission to inspire YOU to look, feel and live your best.

Introduction

One of the best examples of a sustained stress response is that of a race car driver speeding around the track at up to 200 miles per hour. At any moment they could be in a situation which would result in their immediate death. Their heart rates are commonly up from a resting level of 70 beats per minute to 120-150 with short bursts up to their maximum at 180. This involves both physical and psychological stress. It is acute stress (very intense) and short-term (over after the race).

On a day to day basis, we encounter different situations which cause our own personal stress: pressures at work, pressures at home, time pressure, life changes. Our personal stress can result in a similar body reaction as the race car driver, but with 2 major differences: a milder response to stress (low intensity), but longer duration (long-term). Our stress levels, although not as immediately life-threatening as the race car driver's, and less intense, are long-term because we can feel them up to 24 hours a day. This chronic type of stress is the most damaging because it never goes away—and thus wears on the body over time.

Our focus in this book is primarily dealing with chronic stress, its impact on our body, health, and life. Strategies to help you deal with your personal stress issues are discussed, and a personal worksheet area in the back of the book helps you get specific about your plan moving forward.

Best wishes for health and success!

The following are transcripts from a Teleseminar by Dr. Vartabedian and Debi Silber.

Dr. Roy: Hi everybody, I'm Dr. Roy Vartabedian of Nutripoints.com. I'm here with Debi Silber, the Mojo Coach (TheMojoCoach.com). This program is entitled **"How to Ride Your Own Personal Stress Wave and Thrive."**

Debi: Hi everyone. Today we're going to be talking all about how to ride your own personal stress wave and thrive. Let's just dive right in. Dr. Roy, tell us about all the stress we have. What's going on here?

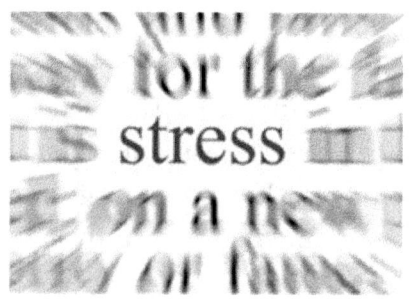

The American Psychological Association found 80% of doctor visits are due to stress, which results in 550 million work days lost each year.

Dr. Roy: Well, Debi we all know that stress is a big problem today, especially in the United States, but in all of the developed countries, and the reason is that there are two big things happening.

One is the pace of society is increasing tremend-ously with all of the technology that we have, with all the information that we're bombarded with, with the internet, with cell phones, every moment there's some sort of information being thrown at you and the changes that can occur because of that happening very quickly with no time in between to bounce back, and your body to rejuvenate itself.

The other thing is that we have a lot less social support than we had years ago when two or three generations lived together, people were more stable, they were more stable with their move-ments, more stable with their jobs and so forth.

We've got more stress. In fact, one stress researcher estimates that we have about a thousand times more stress-producing events in our lifetimes than our great grandparents did.

So we have more stress, but we have less coping mechanisms and less social support to help us deal with it today.

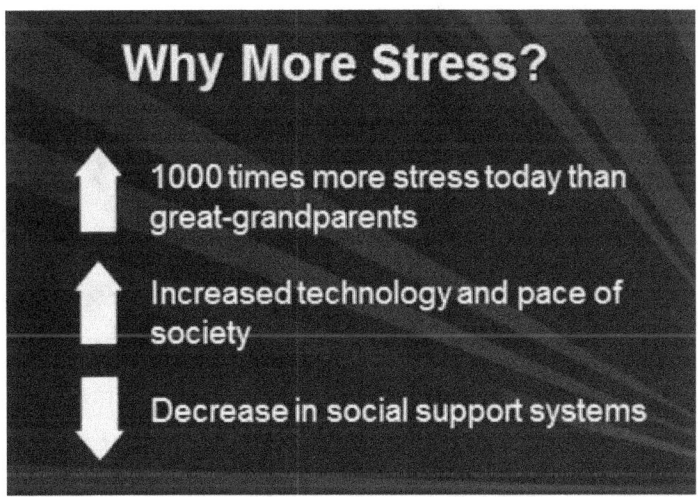

7

AVERAGE STRESS LEVEL BY GENERATION

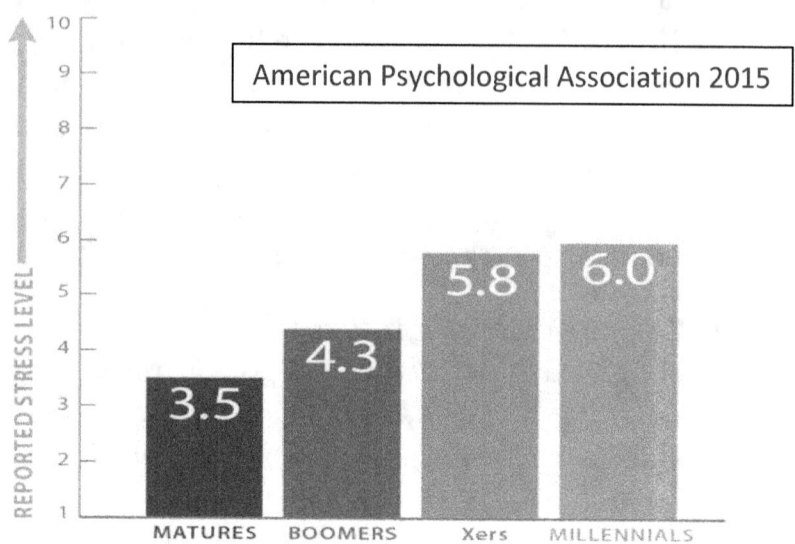

American Psychological Association 2015

REPORTED STRESS LEVEL

| MATURES | BOOMERS | Xers | MILLENNIALS |
| 3.5 | 4.3 | 5.8 | 6.0 |

BASE: ALL QUALIFIED RESPONDENTS 2015 (Echoes/Millennials n=1190; Xers n=649; Boomers n=1130; Matures n=392)

Q605 On a scale of 1 to 10 where 1 means you have "little or no stress" and 10 means you have "a great deal of stress," how would you rate your average level of stress during the past month?

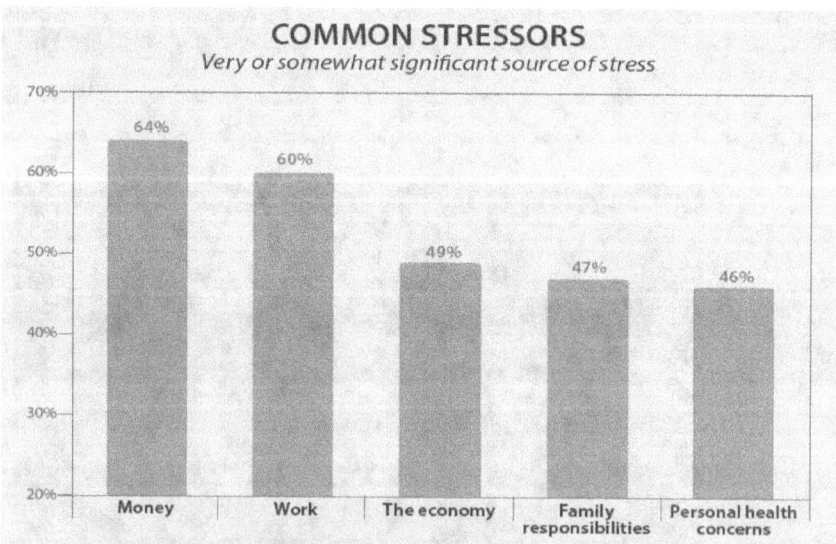

COMMON STRESSORS
Very or somewhat significant source of stress

| Money | Work | The economy | Family responsibilities | Personal health concerns |
| 64% | 60% | 49% | 47% | 46% |

BASE: ALL QUALIFIED RESPONDENTS 2014 (n=3068)

Q625 Below is a list of things people say cause stress in their lives. For each one, please indicate how significant a source of stress it is in your life.

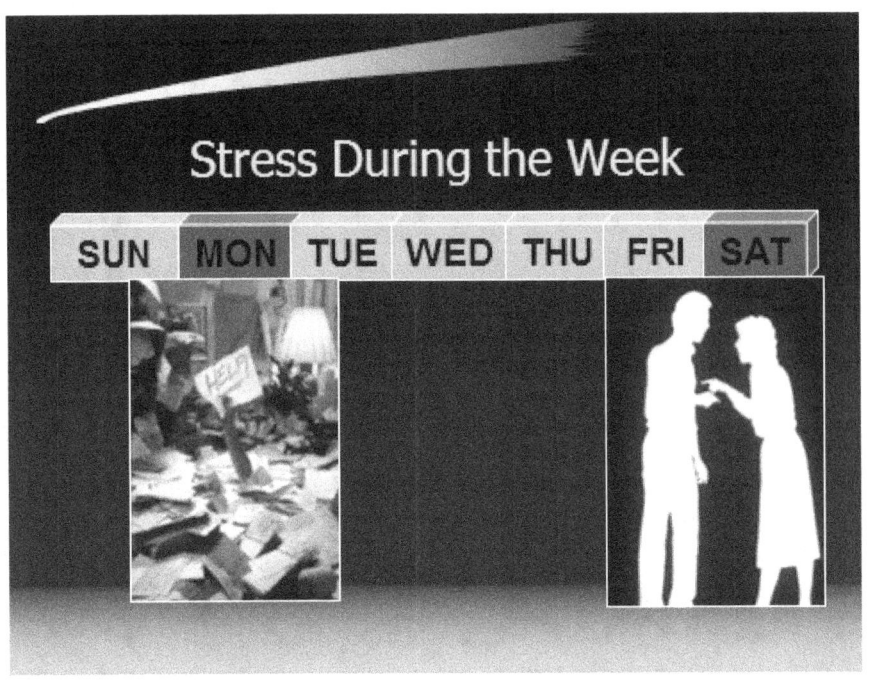

Debi: And what's so interesting is I think so many of us aren't really aware of how our bodies react to stress, and what I'd like to do is just briefly tell everyone what goes on here.

We have two kinds of stress. We have acute stress and chronic stress. With acute stress that's watching cars coming at you and we perceive this as a threat. Your body is designed to keep you safe. It's to keep you safe and to keep you alive.

So let's just say a car's coming at you and we decide that it's a threat to our safety, and again nothing is actually considered a threat to our safety unless we decide it is, but let's just say a car's coming at us. It's a threat to our safety.

Think of what's going to happen here. We're going to have a burst of adrenaline, this surge of hormones and chemicals that flood through our system. We have more blood and oxygen pumping to the heart and lungs. The pupils dilate. With this we get this burst of energy. We jump the curb to safety. That's exactly what's the stress response is designed for—to keep us safe, to keep us alive.

With chronic stress, what happens is this same system is ignited but it's not turned off. So the same system that's designed to protect you over the short term is actually causing huge wear and tear over the long term.

It's sort of like turning the hot water on full blast then walking away. Eventually you're going to run out of hot water. Your body doesn't know and doesn't really care if the stress you feel is real or imagined. So your body is going to react whether a car is coming at you, whether you're feeling the stress of parenting, whether you're feeling the stress of your job, whether your re-living a fight with your own mom ten years ago—it doesn't matter.

If your body perceives it's under stress and there's a threat to your safety, it's going to ignite the stress response, and over time it causes huge wear and tear.

Dr. Roy: Debi that's a great point about how you perceive it is very important. For example, in animals they just respond to a physical threat physically, and they burn up the stress either running away or fighting. But in humans we not only don't do that, most of the time we don't fight, we try to deal with it some other way and it's a psychological stress. But the other thing we do that is different than animals is that we can have imagined fears and imagined stress—things that we worry about that either happened in the past or may not ever happen in the future, and we go through the same stress response.

Mark Twain had a great quote on this. He said, "In my time I've seen a great many troubles—but most of them never happened."

> ## "In my time I've seen a great many troubles—but most of them never happened."
> ## Mark Twain

Debi: It's so true, and I remember reading a book, *Why Zebras Don't Get Ulcers*, by Robert Sapolsky, and because animals don't hold a grudge.

ROBERT M. SAPOLSKY

Author of *A Primate's Memoir*

WHY ZEBRAS DON'T GET ULCERS

The Acclaimed Guide to Stress,
Stress-Related Diseases, and Coping

"One of the best science writers of our time."
—Oliver Sacks

Now Revised and Updated

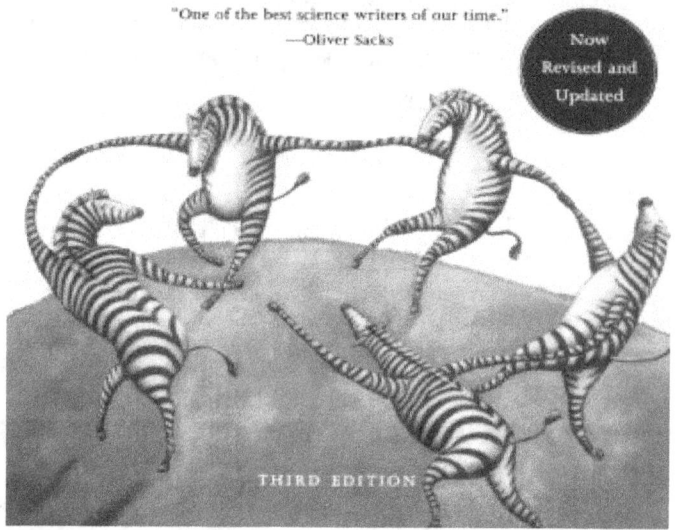

THIRD EDITION

There's not all that afterthought, and that's what keeps that stress response going. I'll tell you years ago when it comes to health and wellness, as a dietitian and trainer, I really thought all you needed was to eat well and exercise—and I was dead wrong! What had happened was I started getting all of these symptoms, illnesses, and diseases that I just attributed to either bad luck, or bad genes.

I can tell you the progression of it: it started with bursitis in my shoulder, couldn't really lift packages, lift my kids. So I had a shot of cortisone in my shoulder. From there I started having just a lot of anxiety and insomnia, started gaining weight, I started breaking out, I started losing my hair.

From there I was getting all kinds of upper respiratory infections and viruses. I was getting sick all the time and that led to starting to have back problems and it got so bad at one point I almost tried to stop driving because I couldn't turn my head to look over my shoulder.

A few doctors said that I had two herniated discs and degenerative disc disease. I had one weighted cartilage that cushions the disc. So they were pressing directly on the nerves. You could imagine that kind of pain, right?

They said surgery was inevitable so that was kind of it. And after that, if that wasn't bad enough, soon after that I developed severe arthritis in my feet. And from the outside they were fine, but x-ray showed again that I had worn away my cartilage, and went to a bunch of doctors and they just said, "Well it's probably from all of your years of running." because I had been a runner.

And you know when that light bulb goes off, I'm thinking about it and I'm saying "Why is it that some people can run into their 70s, and here I could barely walk before my 40th birthday?"

Something clearly wasn't right. I had a feeling there was a link between my stress and my health.

So I had to have surgery because I could barely walk. But I studied to become a whole health coach—and that's a health expert trained to teach how your lifestyle creates health and wellness or illness and disease—and sure enough I found I was like the poster child for stress-related illnesses and conditions, and what I did was sort of this personal experiment, and I slowly changed everything.

And as I did, every single illness, symptom, condition, disease I had—healed, and I went from complete illness to health and complete pain to pain-free living, and really complete misery to joy, and it was truly a result of managing this chronic stress, and when we get a handle on it and take responsibility for the stressors in our lives we can heal mentally, physically and emotionally.

Dr. Roy: That's an amazing story, Debi, because what it really tells you is that stress actually accelerates the whole aging process, and the whole chronic disease process. So you had compressed all that into a short period of time. But the good news is that at any point in time we can stop that process and reverse it, and the body can change and become healthy—because it is constantly replenishing itself, and is constantly replenishing all the different cells and components of the cells so that you can get stronger and stronger.

The nerves can become stronger based on all the different techniques that you use to help you relax and get positive things in your life and so forth, and so at a young age you were having all those problems that most people have later in their life, but you made the dramatic changes and made it reverse.

As you mentioned anxiety, fatigue, depression, insomnia, even muscle tremors, shakiness—all these things are signs and symptoms that you're on the way and then the diseases that are related to them come. Particularly things like heart disease, cancer—because your immune system is depressed, hypertension—because all those hormones being secreted by the adrenal glands are increasing your blood pressure during that fight or flight situation, things like ulcers, colitis and diabetes which is a major, major problem today is caused by stress—because you've got an increase in blood glucose, an increase in cholesterol, and we aren't burning that up.

So it just sits around the pancreas and overloads it. Then you mentioned some allergic type of reaction or allergies can be—the threshold for allergies can go down when you're under stress. A lot of these things start surfacing and when you start feeling those things, they are the signs that you need to make a change.

Debi: You're so right and I think what happens is we are so busy and this is part of the stress. We're so busy that we don't pay attention to these symptoms and we just—well like I said, we attribute it to either just bad luck or bad genes and in not paying attention to them we're not doing anything to correct them.

And it's one thing after another after another until it manifests itself into this illness or disease, because at some point you're going to need to pay attention and your body's speaking to you and it's going to get you to listen no matter what it takes.

Stress-Related Diseases

- Heart disease
- Cancer
- Diabetes
- Hypertension
- Hyperlipidemia
- Allergies
- Asthma
- Obesity
- Headaches
- Depression
- GI conditions
- Skin conditions
- Insomnia
- Drug abuse
- Arrhythmias
- Mental Disorders

But one of the biggest things that I noticed also was you had mentioned with your immune system— your immune system is like this internal army. It protects its borders against invasion when that army is strong and when that immune system is strong.

When it's suppressed, which is because of stress, that's when—it's almost like that army is fast asleep and we're susceptible to all of these viral and bacterial invasions and that's when we find when that we get sick all the time.

I had read a couple of studies where they studied students who were cramming for exams. Such a huge amount of students would get sick right after the exams, or if you're planning for a big event and then there's that pimple right on your nose on the big day.

Well because your skin is acting up, and so much of it has to do with the stress that we're under. Every thought we have contains a chemical and a hormone that will either nurture, support and heal or cause physical, emotional and mental wear and tear.

Dr. Roy: Right. If you have the good hormones like the endorphins that are stimulated from exercise and just generally good things happening in your life, your body will start secreting these positive hormones which actually have a healing effect on the body as you mentioned, Debi.

So that's the problem. So what do we do about it? I've developed a 3-step process (3 stress-shields) that I think really hits all the major components of how we can deal with stress and it works something like this.

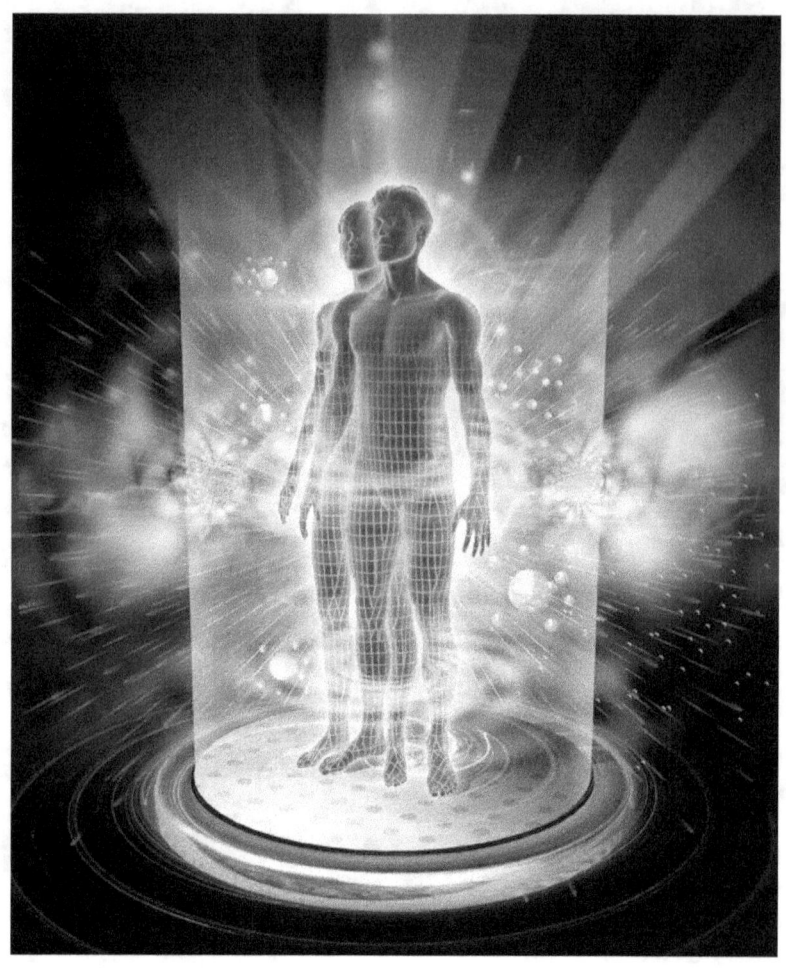

Number one is we hit it from the source. We try to decrease the number of stressors in our life, or try to spread them out. That's one way.

Number two is to change our perception and attitude of stress so that the inevitable stress that gets to us does not affect is because we're blocking it by not perceiving it in a negative way.

Number three is to use coping mechanisms to help you deal with the stress that still gets through even those two filters.

So what I'd like to do Debi, and get your input as well, is go through some of the specifics in those three areas.

Debi: And what I would encourage everyone to do is start writing these down. The first one that Dr. Roy mentioned was to decrease your number of stressors. Take a minute here and think of the stressors, think of the things that actually cause you stress, what's really providing that stress for you and some things that may come up would be—and it's always—it's things that we take on.

I mean this is all self-induced. We have a choice with everything that we do, so maybe this could be the way we're handling a relationship that we have, and we're not protecting ourselves from the mental and the emotional, and again the physical wear and tear.

So maybe there's a person that's triggering you to feel this stress. Maybe it's a boring unfulfilling job, or you're working for someone that's just—you're feeling the stress from that person.
You're having a rough time with your kids and maybe it's coming from that place. Those are a few. Dr. Roy from you, any stressors that you...?

Dr. Roy: Those are great. I think the first thing Debi is to list what are the stressful things, and then what I'm going to do is give you some ways that you can deal with those, and as I give them look through those maybe five top ones that relate to these specific ways.

Now the things that are on your list that you can either cut out or change somehow—these are the things that I'm going to look at first. For example, one thing that you can do to decrease the number of stressors is to prioritize, and then don't sweat the small stuff.

We've all heard that before. Don't sweat the small stuff. A lot of people get caught up in details, and those details take a lot of time and energy, and then you don't have the time and energy for the things that are really important to you.

So maybe there are some things that you can just cut out and it's not going to make any difference at all. Look down the road maybe one year, two years, five years down the road—is this going to make any difference at all? If it's not, then maybe you can cut it out and focus on the things that are high priority to you.

Another way we can do it is maybe you have a lot of these things that are happening one after another, or as you're looking at your schedule during the day or during the week or during the month, you see that you've got two things happening here and you don't want to put another thing in right on the same day or near it.

Try to spread out those very eventful times in your life. Of course there's going to be the unexpected where things come in and throw things all of out of kilter. But build a little time into your schedule.

There was one doctor. He said he would always build one or two fictitious patients into his schedule during the day to give him a little buffer there so when the unexpected came, it wasn't going to be a big stress!

Another is we can learn to say no. If we're pleasers or want to help people, it's a great thing but if you're a nurturer, a lot of times you can get so drained and you need to look out for yourself first, and you need to learn to say no when your limit has been passed—and you're the only one that knows that.

A lot of times we compare ourselves to other people. We say "Well they're doing this, so I should be able to do it." No. You're the one that knows how it's affecting you the most, so you are in control and only you can make that decision.

The other thing is just don't be available and accessible 7 days a week, 24 hours a day. We need a day off during the week. We need little breaks during the day and we need our sleep at night.

So these are all ways that you can decrease the number of stressors in your life or spread them out somehow.

Debi: And I would tell you that those points are so important and even something like to say no. If I tell you how many times throughout my practice— I've actually worked with moms on the most effective ways for them to say no, because we're taught that we're just supposed to give endlessly at the expense of everything.

We think that we're perceived as being nice or being a team player or just going along with things, but the problem is we're just depleting ourselves and causing huge stress, and just really not staying true to our priorities and our values— just because we haven't found the right way to say no.

So whether it's "Thank you so much for the offer. I have a little bit too much on my plate right now. If things change I'll let you know." –whatever the words are, it's crucial to find the right phrase so you can just say no.

Dr. Roy: And don't feel guilty about it, because you need what you need so that you can give to other people. We've all heard that before, but it's so true as a mom especially. Debi, working with moms I can see that because there are so many things to do and they have to give so much that they really have to look out for themselves.

But we all do as well. Everybody has to do it at some point. So be in tune when you're getting those symptoms and realize that you need to take some time for yourself or do some of the things that you enjoy.

Now if you look at your list of the 5 most stressful things in your life, there are going to be some things that you can't cut out, but maybe you can change your perception or attitude towards the stressful events.

Let me give you an example. Let's say that there is somebody that's very irritating in your life. Let's think about that one person in our life that is just so irritating, we don't want to be around them, we always have a problem with them, we want to avoid them. There's something wrong with that person.

Now let's say that somebody comes up to you confidentially and tells you that this person has a brain tumor and the tumor is growing. There's no surgery, there's nothing that can be done about it. Some of you might say "I hope the tumor grows faster!"

But let's just say you're going to be nice about it and realize that maybe that there is a situation causing the bad behavior. You might be more understanding towards that person now. You changed your perception just because somebody told you that fact about them and now you might be more patient and more understanding around that person because you understand why their behavior is a certain way.

When it comes down to it everybody behaves the way they behave for a certain reason. We don't know what that reason is and maybe we have nothing to do with it and there's nothing we can do to change it, but if we can change our perception about that person based on a possibility of some cause of it, that might be one way to change our perception of a person.

Debi: And that's such a great point. We can't change anyone else, and I've seen this and I'm sure you have too so many times, and this is a huge source of frustration and stress for a lot of people because they think they can change someone.

The only person we can change, and that's difficult enough, is ourselves. So if we can find a different way to look at someone—using that example that you've mentioned, or even whatever it's going to take for us, and I'll suggest as well maybe imagining this coat of armor you have around you that no one can penetrate with their hurtful words.

Or even—this may sound a little silly but if there was let's say a monkey jabbering at you. You wouldn't really be offended or hurt or angry about what the monkey said because it's just a monkey right?

Dr. Roy: That's a great point.

Debi: Well maybe what we need to do is sort of envision this person that's harmful, hurtful person as just like a monkey and those same words now won't have the same effect on us, because obviously they're experiencing their own pain and we just need to change our perspective so it doesn't cause us that wear and tear.

Dr. Roy: That's a great analogy, and we need to be thick-skinned.

Dr. Robert Elliot, who's a big stress researcher, wrote books on the subject. He said, why don't we just try to react a 1 or a 2 on a scale of 1 to 10 instead of a 9 or a 10? If you think about it you can control how you react to it. So you can try to tone it down.

IS IT WORTH DYING FOR?

How to Make
Stress Work
for You—
Not Against You

"I have the utmost admiration for Dr. Eliot's book,
as I have for the man himself."
—Norman Cousins, author of *Anatomy of an Illness*

by Dr. Robert S. Eliot
and Dennis L. Breo

Introduction by Michael E. DeBakey, M.D.

Another thing that he did is an experiment with people—remember the first video games that came out? It was that pong game where you'd hit the ping pong ball back and forth on the computer, and he would hook people up to a monitor measuring their blood pressure, their heart rate, and their total peripheral resistance—the resistance of the blood flow through the small capillaries in the body.

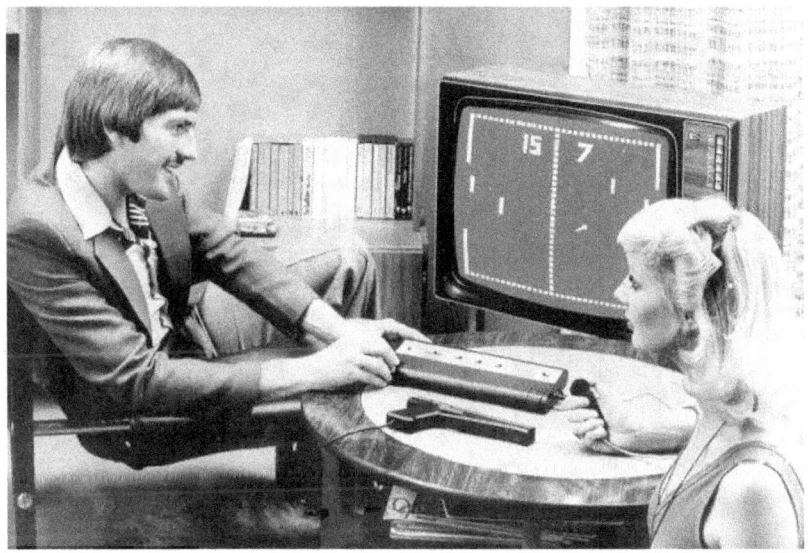

What he found is when they were winning the game, everything was fine. The blood pressure would go up slightly, the total peripheral resistance would go down, the blood vessels would open up and the heart rate would go up slightly, and everything was fine.

But then he turned the dial so that it got harder and harder, to the point that they could not win the game. Now how did that person respond in that situation if they were what he calls a hot reactor? What they did is they said "I'm going to beat this game if it kills me!"

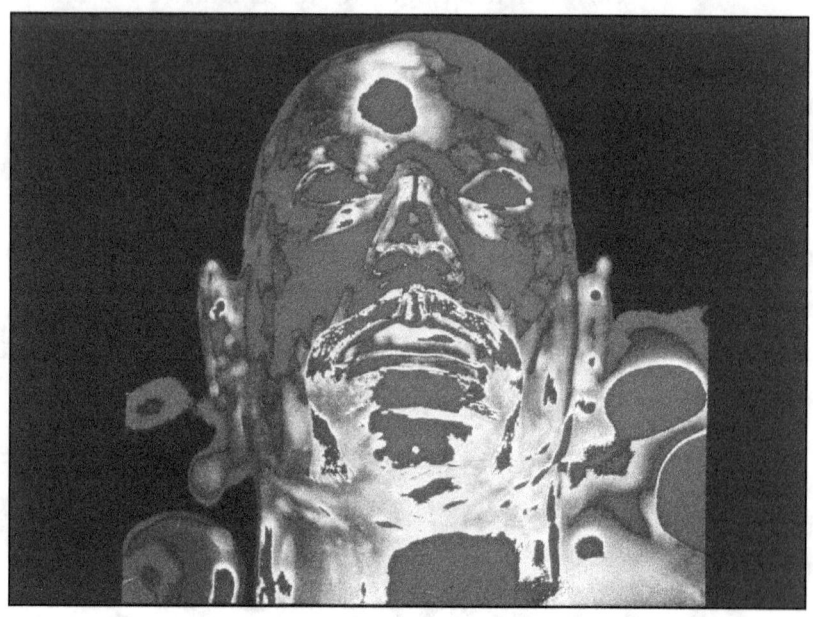

And what it does is actually "kills" them, if not in reality. But what it does is if they were a hot reactor, he can predict that they're going to have a major cardiovascular catastrophe in the next 5 to 6 months based on his test. What happens is the heart rate goes up a lot, the blood pressure goes up a lot and the blood vessels clamp down and less blood can actually be pumped while the heart is trying to pump more blood to increase blood flow.

So if you're in a no win situation what do you do? Do you bang your head against the wall and keep trying or do you back off and change your perception, your attitude and your reaction to it because like you said, Debi, you can only change yourself. You can't change anything else or any other people in many cases.

So if there's nothing you can do about, it all you can change is your reaction to it.

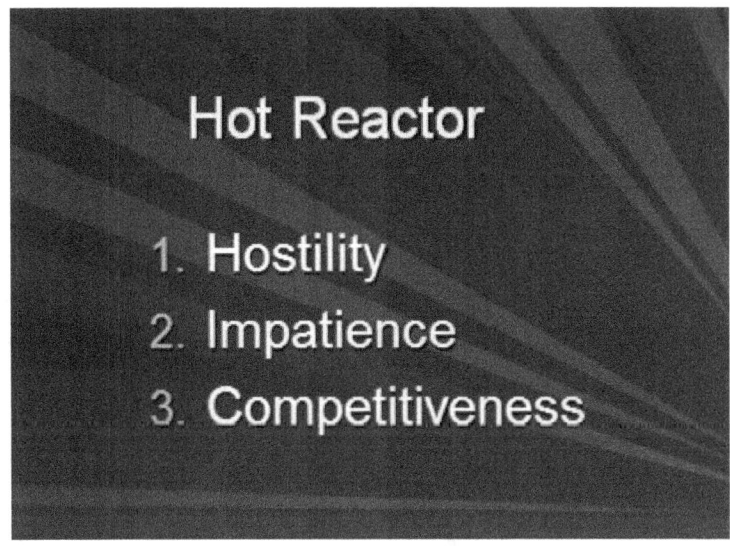

Hot Reactor

1. Hostility
2. Impatience
3. Competitiveness

Debi: And a point I just really want to get across again—this is what's so amazing and the gift that we all have, this is within our control. I think what happens is we're so used to handing over our power. We go from expert to expert and guru to guru and doctor to doctor saying help me, heal me, fix me.

But the reality is when we take responsibility for our thoughts, our behaviors, our actions, our habits—that's where we become empowered and inspired, and that's when we can make these changes because these are things that are absolutely 100% within our control.

We've just been reacting habitually, but through this awareness we can change those habits that are causing these illnesses and symptoms and conditions, diseases. Truly, and it creates a much higher quality of life than what we've been living.

Dr. Roy: That's very true Debi. Thanks for that point, and let's just say that one of the things that you're worrying about on your list of 5 things is something that's going to happen in the future.

Now we do this all the time. We're thinking about what's going to happen, what could happen, what's the worst case scenario and so forth, but what we have to ask ourselves is this: "Are the things I'm worrying about based on reality or is it just something that will probably never happen?"

And the other thing is to remember Mark Twain's quote about most of the things never happen. It's been estimated that 97% of the things that we worry about never happen, and the 3% that do aren't as bad as we thought they were going to be!

So that's a lot of wasted energy and the only thing you can do is change your perception and your attitude about it, and turn off that worry and have the peace that you deserve by not worrying about it because it's not going to happen and it probably won't be as bad.

Debi: And think of what you can do with that mental energy and that extra time if you were to stop worrying and think of the space you've created to do something so constructive and so positive and so proactive.

Look at the difference. Look what a difference your life would be.

Dr. Roy: That's for sure. It's kind of like wasting money. It's a bank account and you've got so much and you've got to spend it wisely. I believe that we all have a certain amount of energy that we have in our whole lifetime, and if we're very efficient with it we'll live longer and we'll be at a higher level of wellness along the way.

Now let's take a look at those five things that are stressful to you again and maybe you've cut out everything that you could in there. You tried to change your perception. We can do the best that we can.

Obviously if there's something like a life change, there's a death in the family or some tragic accident, some things that are out of our control, we can't cut that stress out and we can change our attitude about it as much as we want, but still a lot of that stress is going to filter through just because that event is so much of a shock to you.

The third thing that you can do is use all of the coping mechanisms that you have at your disposal to help you deal with that stress, to help you burn off that stress and to help you get rid of it so that your body can be as strong as possible.

Debi, the first one that I think is the most important way to cope with stress is to use exercise because exercise is nature's tranquilizer. It actually burns up all of those stress related hormones and chemicals that have been secreted so that you can fully relax, because if those hormones and chemicals are still there it's hard to "psych" yourself into relaxing.

Exercise will burn that up. It will also put a governor effect on stress. Studies have shown that it'll put a governor effect on the body's stress response when you have stress again in the future. So I feel that exercise is the number one key for coping with stress. A research study with fit and unfit school teachers showed this.

Fitness Level	Resting	Teaching
Sedentary	75	105
Fit	60	65

Debi: Definitely and I agree and you're flooding yourself with these endorphins that have been shown to heal, support and nourish. It's interesting; I read a study recently where psychologists were actually taking some of their patients on walks. It's called "walking therapy" because they are seeing that the benefits were so much more significant when they were actually using those natural resources of the endorphins that we have.

Dr. Roy: Definitely. They definitely need that. There are a lot of psychological issues that these people need to go through in therapy, but just plain old burning up the stress is going to help them have a more positive outlook on life, which is going to help feed back everything in a positive way. So it's a great thing to do if you're feeling depressed or stressed. Get those hormones, those endorphins up there through exercise.

The number two way that I feel, and I am sure you agree with this one Debi, is to get the best nutrition that you can to help strengthen your body to handle the inevitable stress that you're going to have. Now remember that nutrition not only fuels the body by giving it energy and the right kind of energy, but it actually helps build and rebuild the body on a cellular level because your body is constantly replacing cells and replacing the components of cells, and the quality of what you're eating is so important because your body is transforming itself every day, every week, every month, every year and if you put in good material—not just the fuel but the building blocks, the material your body can actually recreate itself and become stronger so that you can withstand the inevitable stress that you're going to have much better.

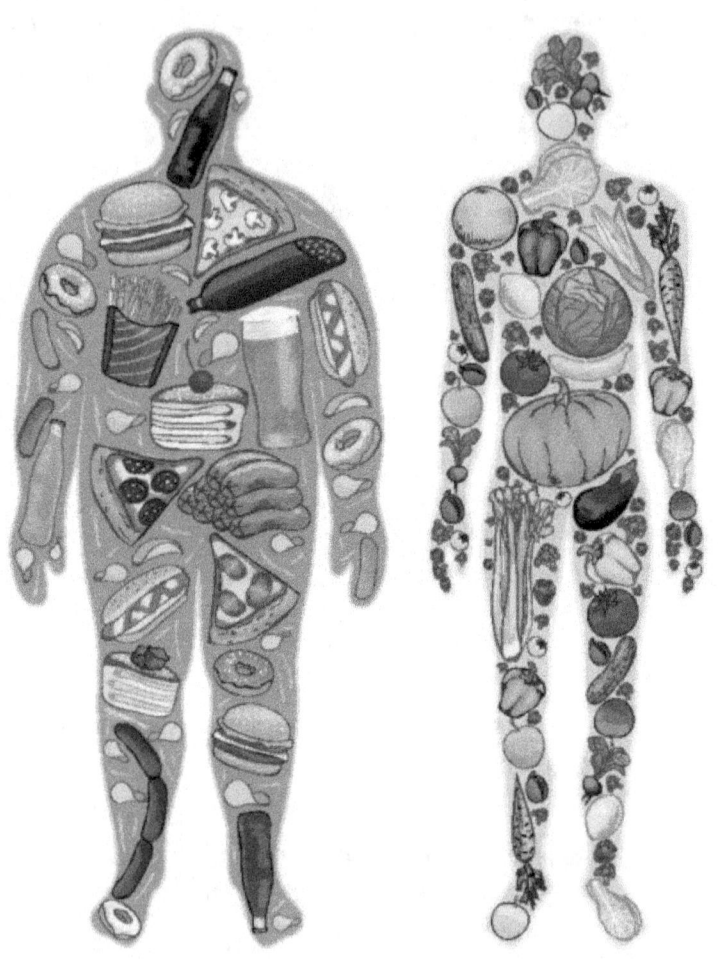

Debi: Definitely and also healthy foods are boosting your immune system, which is suppressed with stress. So it's a proven way to just really build it back up.

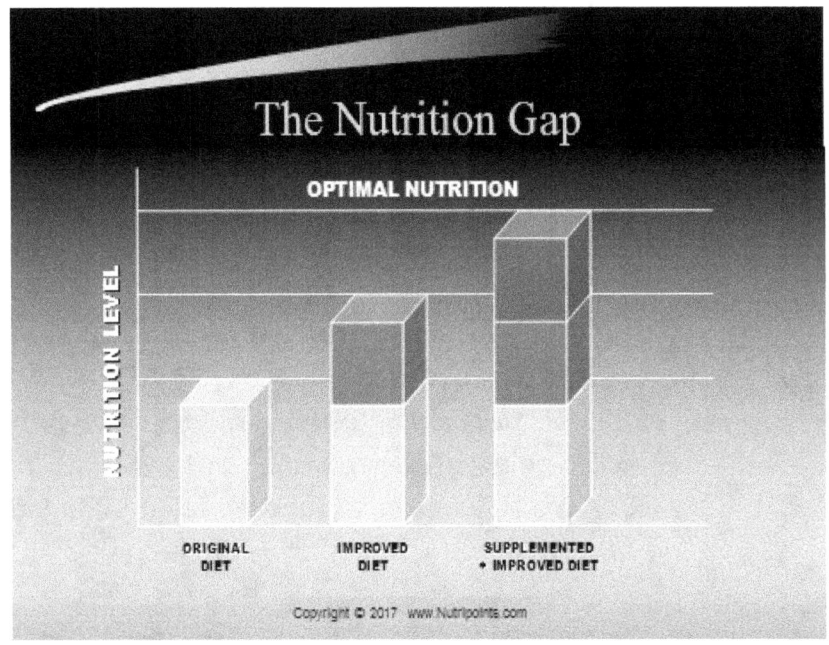

The Nutrition Gap

OPTIMAL NUTRITION

NUTRITION LEVEL

ORIGINAL DIET | IMPROVED DIET | SUPPLEMENTED + IMPROVED DIET

Copyright © 2017 www.Nutripoints.com

I just want to touch back on exercise for a minute. Besides the endorphins that you're giving yourself that you're flooding yourself with through exercise, what's also so helpful with exercise is you're doing something that you're controlling. When we're so overwhelmed, when we have so much stress on us, a big part of that is feeling that our lives are out of control, and here is where exercise is so powerful because we're physically doing something to take that control back and that is a great way to lessen the stress.

Dr. Roy: Very good. Thank you, Debi, for that. Another way that I think is very important is to use water. Now we're talking about drinking water, drinking pure water, getting enough water to flush out the wastes out of our system because our bodies are at least

70% water and so we need to hydrate. We need to keep as much water in the body as the body needs because when it gets low, our performance goes down physically, all the chemical reactions do not work as well. Our kidneys have to work harder to filter the blood and so forth, so it's important to drink enough water.

Studies have found that we need about 1/3 more water than our thirst tells us. So, if you drink a little bit more than you actually feel like drinking, you're going to be getting closer to what you need. Now it's also important to use water on the outside of the body to cleanse and also to help you relax.

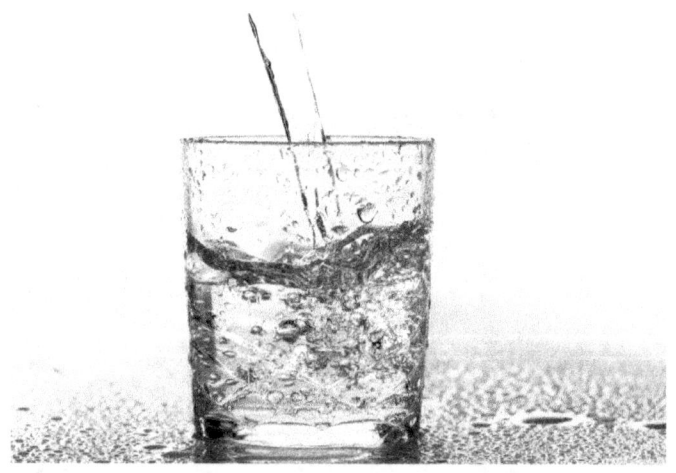

I know for myself the best thing for me when I get stressed out is to take a hot bath. It just melts the stress away, or a Jacuzzi or whirlpool, whatever form of it that you like, but the heat and the water together, the combination is very relaxing. So water inside the body to cleanse, and outside the body to help you relax.

Debi: And I would just add to that one when we are dehydrated we're also very tired. It's a huge sign of fatigue. What happens is we get extremely, extremely tired. Stress is causing that fatigue as well, so by rehydrating yourself you're actually increasing your energy and just helping to deal with the stress in that way as well.

Dr. Roy: Very good. Now extending that a little bit as far as the relaxation that we get from the water would be to practice relaxation techniques, what we call "progressive muscle relaxation." There are a lot of tapes that are out that help you start at one part of your body and mentally go through and relax you're whole body to the point where you just feel totally relaxed. There is also biofeedback which you can do where you hook yourself up either with a machine that you use at home or with a therapist where you can measure your heart rate and your blood pressure, and you actually mentally try and relax, and when you see that what you've done mentally—it's kind of like practicing how to do control over your body to relax it. When you feel it doing it, you get the feedback from the machines, and then you do that over and over again so that you can actually control more fully your relaxation process.

Now another thing that is really relaxing would be sunlight. How many people that you've seen that have been stressed that are out there on the beach? There is actually a physiological reaction where sunlight will reduce some of the catecholamines, some of the chemicals and hormones that are secreted by stress in the body. So there actually is a physiological response to sunlight.

Now, of course, we need to make sure that we don't get too much sunlight for skin cancer and so forth, and screen out those burning rays. That is one thing. I read a book on sunlight, the whole book was on sunlight, and all of the different benefits of it. People are really afraid of the sun nowadays, but there are a lot of actual positive benefits to getting some sunlight, maybe 15-20 minutes a day of good sunlight. Not too much to prevent the burning and so forth but at least something because a lot of us stay indoors almost all day. What this creates is an artificial environment and we need that natural sunlight on our skin and through our eyes. If you're wearing sunglasses all of the time you're not getting that natural sunlight, so get a little bit of natural sunlight each day.

Now we're finding that vitamin D is so important. Many people have low levels of vitamin D and the sunlight actually helps build that in our bodies.

Debi: You know what and I would suggest as well? Everybody has something that really relaxes them. It's a very personal individual thing so maybe for some it's a walk in nature. For others it's playing with puppies, for others it's actually cleaning. They might find that very therapeutic.

Taking a walk through a bookstore or just having time alone, just lighting some candles or just reading or journaling, meditating, listening to music, whatever it is. It is really important to find out what your personal stress-reliever is and then make sure it's available. Make sure you do that when you do feel stressed.

Dr. Roy: Right, a lot of us are working so much or we're so busy that we haven't even done some of our 5 favorite things in life. Think about what are your favorite things and how long has it been since you've done any of them, or how often has it been since you've done them. Is it walking on the beach, or like Debi said what is it for you that is your favorite thing? Those are the things that are going to rejuvenate you specifically, and that is what you need to do. It might even be cleaning because it helps you express yourself, burn up some energy and you feel good when it's all done.

Another way to cope with stress is to express your feelings. This is a big factor. What they've found is that people who hold their feelings in are more likely to have high blood pressure because all of those feelings are bottled up, and it's a way of releasing those chemicals and hormones in a positive way by expressing those feelings.

It's really important to do that and one study actually showed that people that cry a lot, when they're crying they actually did an analysis of the tears and found that some of the stress-related hormones and chemicals are actually being secreted through tears. So you're actually physiologically reducing your stress.

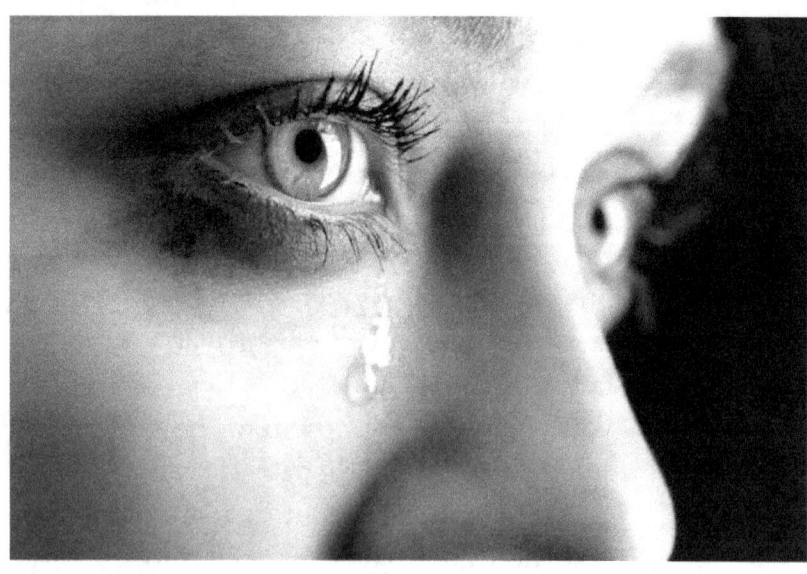

If you have some feelings, and I'm not saying go out and just get angry or something like that. What I am saying is if you have feelings and you need to talk to somebody about something maybe even start by just writing it out. Maybe that is enough to do it. A lot of times we need to directly express our feelings in some way so that we don't have it all staying inside of us. It actually can cause a lot of problems. It can cause the stress response at a chronic low level over a long period of time if we don't do that.

Debi: It's so true, and the one thing I would add to that is when you're expressing your feelings—and it's such a great thing to do—what you really want to avoid is judging those feelings because you see that is where we get into trouble. Because if we're feeling something and then we start saying, "Well, I shouldn't be feeling this and why do I feel that?" then you get angry or upset with yourself, that is where the chronic stress now is kicking in, where instead if you sort of experiencing those feelings— anger, frustration and look at it more from a curious standpoint. You're looking at it through curiosity instead of judgment. Then you're sort of saying, OK, this is what I'm feeling, and then you have an opportunity to do something more positive with it instead of just berating yourself and being angry with yourself and feeding into the stress.

Dr. Roy: Very good, very good. Thank you, Debi. The last thing that has been shown to help people cope with stress that I wanted to mention is group support and membership to groups. What they found is people that are isolated, out there all by themselves, that don't have any kind of family, friends, or group associations; they are much more susceptible to stress than people that do have good family support. Or even if you don't have that, at least you could have a good friendship network or at least one good friend. Hopefully, it's your spouse or your significant other, but other friends are important as well.

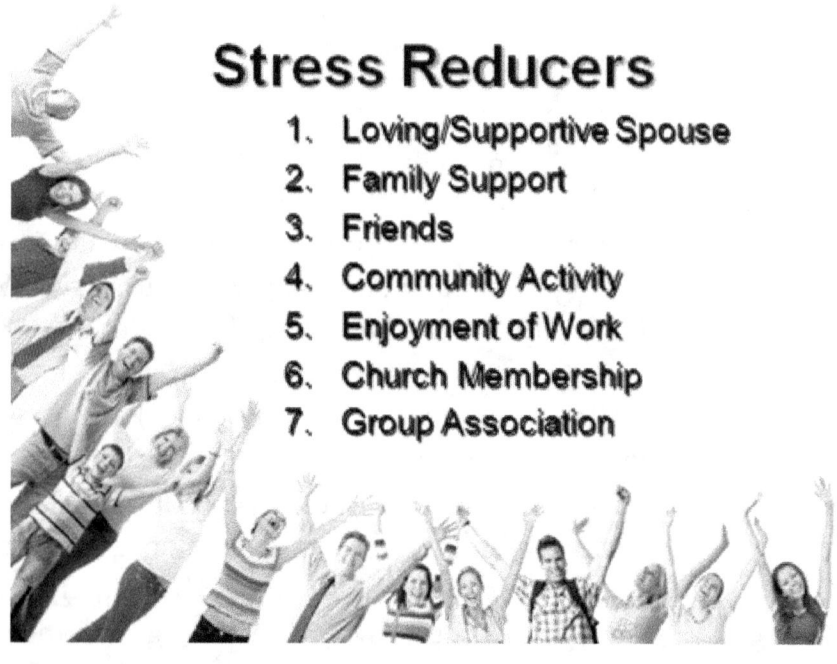

Stress Reducers
1. Loving/Supportive Spouse
2. Family Support
3. Friends
4. Community Activity
5. Enjoyment of Work
6. Church Membership
7. Group Association

Then group association, because what happens is as you identify with other people, share and express things, a lot of times it's part of that expressing of your feelings—but it's also sharing and getting ideas from other people and knowing that other people are going through the same thing that you're going through, or have been through the same thing that you're going through right now, and they can actually help you.

You know when we've all gone through a certain situation; we're more understanding and helpful to other people who go through that same situation. If we have this network with other people whether its family, friends or group, that is going to help us be stronger and withstand a lot more stress.

Debi: That is so true and that is actually why rejection and isolation is so painful. These are basic needs that we have. We have a need to feel a sense of connectedness and that is why those feelings are just as hurtful as they are. There were a few studies out. One I remember was about how they did a study with cancer patients. They separated the two groups—one that had support and one that didn't have support.

The ones that had support had a remission 18 months longer than the others with no other differences other than the support that they had. A part of that is that support, that feeling of connectedness, actually strengthens your immune system. So it's boosting you physically and preventing the invasion of the bacteria, viruses and just strengthening you up physically, mentally and emotionally. So it's powerful; it's really powerful to have that support and that feeling of connectedness around you.

Dr. Roy: So what you're doing, really, is you're turning off the negative hormones and trying to limit the negative hormones from stress and trying to reverse those and increase the positive hormones that are connected with all of the things that we're talking about.

Debi: Absolutely and it's just from everything that we've spoken about so far—these are all things within our control. Even when we just touched on the idea of support, we have people in our lives all of the time. Some are nurturing and supportive and loving and then we have those toxic relationships that are more destructive.

You know those people who are negative, judgmental, critical, pessimistic—think about how you feel when you're spending time with one group as opposed to another. It's a choice. What would benefit us physically as well as mentally and emotionally would be to spend more time with the people who are actually physically good for us and limit our time, and even if we need to cut the ties, with the ones who are damaging mentally and physically and emotionally.

Dr. Roy: Yes and if you're a fix-it type of person like Debi was saying, you keep trying to fix that person so you can get along with them, but all you can do is change yourself and change your environment so that they're not around you. If you have the same situation over and over again, you could be having a great day and then that person comes into your life and it ruins your whole day, you can't sleep, you're thinking about it over and over and over again, you need to avoid that person and that situation because there is no way you can fix somebody else that doesn't want to be fixed.

Debi: Absolutely! We're talking about really controlling our perceptions and our perspectives. I will just give you this example because this is something everyone can relate to. Let's take traffic. The traffic is a situation that we all know and we've all experienced. It's the same situation for all of us.

Let's say we're in the middle lane. You look over into your left lane and you can see someone catching up on phone calls, relaxing, spending some quiet time before they get home and really just taking advantage of that quiet time.

Take a look over into your right lane and here you may find someone banging on the steering wheel and cursing and sort of drowning in this sea of stress-induced hormones. Now it's the same situation for both, but the way they've chosen to handle it is entirely different. This is what we are able to control. It's a choice.

Dr. Roy: And that leads into some of the studies that were done with people that had what they called a "hardy personality," Debi. People that were under the same amount of stress as everybody else were in the group but some people could withstand 2-3 times more stress than the others and didn't get sick. They had more stress and they didn't get sick. They had what they called a "hardy personality."

They had a resistance to stress, and using some of the principles that we talked about you could incorporate that into your being and yourself.

Hardy Personality

1. Openness to Change
2. Feeling of Involvement
3. Sense of Control

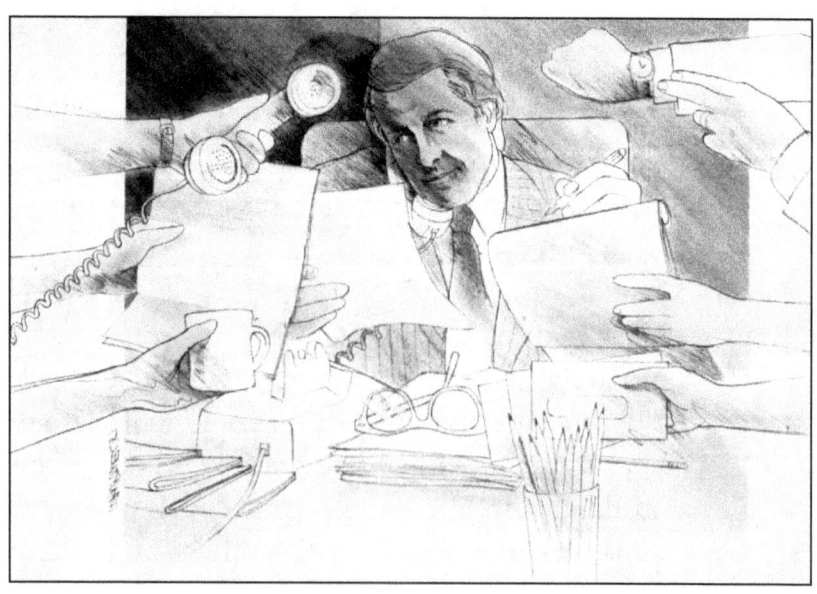

Well, the title of this is "How to Ride Your Own Personal Stress Wave and Thrive." I want to give you an analogy and kind of a system that you could look at to do that. There is a book that was written by Kriegel and Kriegel, Robert Kriegel and Marilyn Kriegel, both PhD's, and what they came up with is a thing called the "C Zone." The "C Zone" is what they call the little groove that you want to be in to be Committed, Confident and in Control of your life.

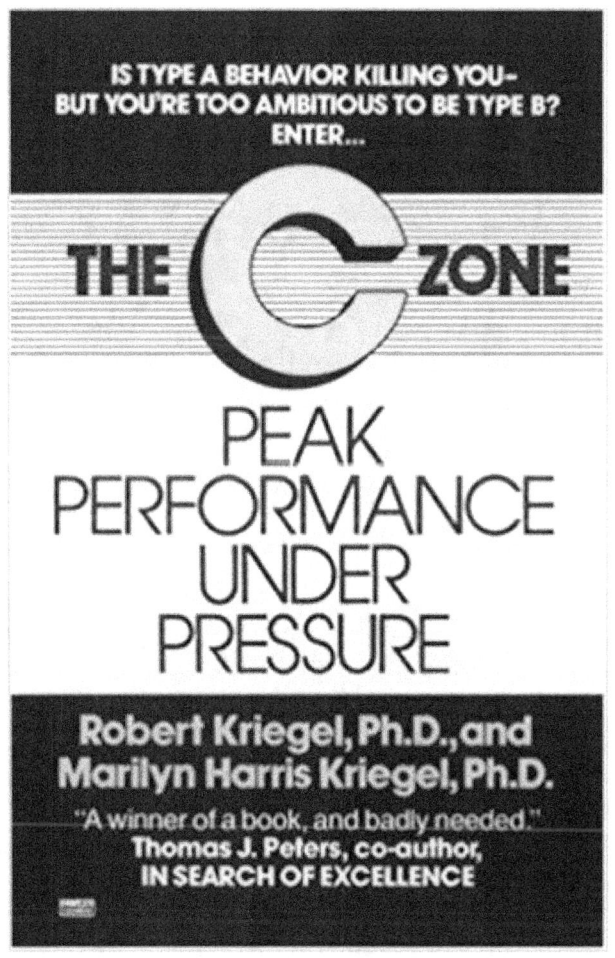

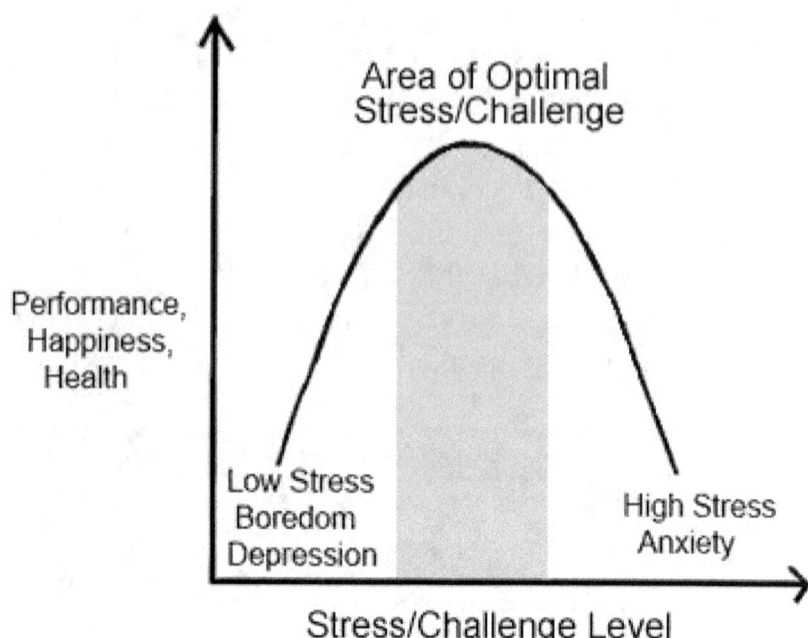

Here is the way it works. All of us have challenges in our life and then we try to overcome those challenges and master them, whether it's our job, at home, with people or whatever we're doing in life. We have the challenges. Now if we have too many challenges and try to take on too many things at once we get into the "panic zone." Now some people aren't on that end of the scale. They are not having enough challenges like the beach bums or something like that. Nothing against the beach; I love the beach!

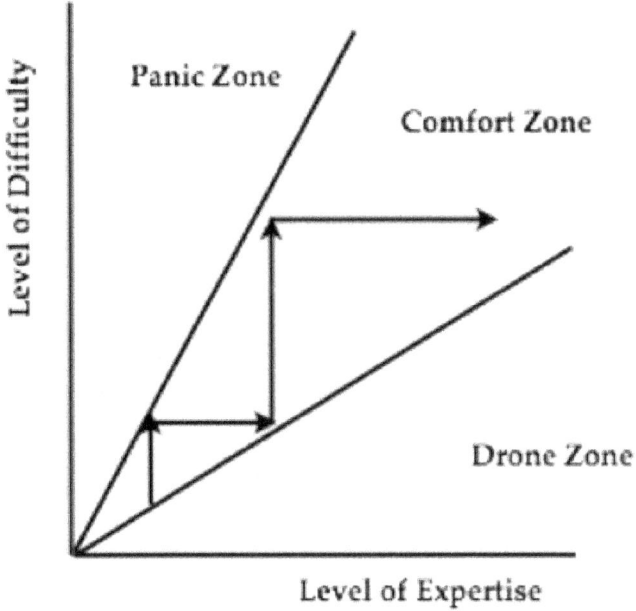

If you have no challenge in your life and you're mastering everything in your life, you get bored. So the key is to try and design our lives in a way so that we have time to master that challenge before we take on new challenges. Not that you can only do one thing at a time, but get to the level of challenges in your life that you can control, so that you can go between mastering those and moving onto other challenges. Going between mastery and challenging yourself so that you're riding that wave that is in the "comfort zone" for you, not the "panic zone" or the "drone zone," but the "C Zone," the comfort zone. Not too comfortable—a little bit of challenge and then you master it. That's I think the balance that we need, Debi.

Debi: Definitely! I think it was Eleanor Roosevelt who said, "Do something that scares you every day." Because if anything is going to break you through that comfort zone, which is really getting out of this place of where we are, where we spend our time if it's not working for us, we need to just challenge ourselves enough to get into the next level or get into something that is more fulfilling, more satisfying, more enriching or rewarding. To do that you do need to burst a little bit past that comfort zone and it will be scary, but it's like you said finding that balance of what feels okay but still makes things exciting for you.

Dr. Roy: And then say no. If you have a lot of other challenges that are coming up, say no to those new ones so that you can keep working on the one or the ones that are important to you that you're working on right now. Try to keep it at a level that you can control.

It's easier said than done, but at least if we know that is what we're trying to do and trying to design it that way, then we can move towards that without just being totally out of control and not knowing where we're going or where we're at.

Debi: That is a very important point.

Dr. Roy: Well everybody, I would encourage you to take your worksheets, and go through those and fill in any of the areas that you haven't. Go through those 5 top stressors and try to use all of those techniques on them and see if you can eliminate the effects of that stress and turn those negative hormones and chemicals into positive ones that will help give you a high level of wellness, more energy, lower some of your risk factors for disease and definitely get rid of all of those symptoms of stress that you might have.

Debi: Everyone, I want to thank you so much for joining us. This is Debi Silber with Dr. Roy Vartabedian. For more information on both of us and what we have to offer, go to either www.Nutripoints.com or www.TheMojoCoach.com.

It's been our pleasure. Take advantage of these CDs and of these worksheets. Listen to them again. Re-read your notes again and really take advantage of finding out what's been causing, what's been going on in your life and then working slowly but specifically towards a better way.

Dr. Roy: Thank you, Debi. It's been great doing this with you, and I wish all of you the best luck, and the best at using all of these techniques to help you in your life and your lifestyle.

Debi: Definitely! Thank you so much. Bye-bye.

Content Summary

Causes of Stress Today:

1. Increased pace of society with no time to recover from multiple stressful events
2. Decreased social support systems to help us naturally deal with stress

The Stress Response:

1. Acute stress—a short-term response to a one-time dangerous event
2. Chronic stress—a long-term sustained low level of stress related to an ongoing issue which can lead to chronic disease
3. If we perceive something as stressful, our bodies will go through the same real stress response, whether the threat is real or imagined
4. Chronic stress accelerates the aging process and is the main type of stress we need to address today

Your Personal Stressors:

1. Write down the top 5 stressful things in your life today
2. Identify those you could decrease or eliminate
3. Identify those you might be able to change your attitude about positively
4. Identify those you could use coping mechanisms to deal with the stress

3-Point Plan to Deal with Stress:

Decrease the number of stressors
1) prioritize, and don't sweat the small stuff
2) spread out changes and leave time in between
3) learn to say "No."
4) take breaks during the day, week, and month

Change your attitude and perception of stress
1) you can't change another person—only your perception of that person
2) if you can't change a situation or event, change your perception of that situation or event
3) learn to be thick-skinned
4) moderate your reactions to stress, react 1 or 2 instead of 9 or 10
5) be flexible—don't have a "win at all costs" mentality
6) evaluate: are the things you're worrying about based on reality?

Use Coping Mechanisms to Deal with Inevitable Stress
1) exercise to burn up the chemical effects of stress and moderate the stress response
2) eat high nutrient density foods like fruits and vegetables to strengthen the body and immune system
3) drink water to flush out wastes (inside body) and relax the body (outside body).
4) use progressive muscle relaxation, biofeedback, massage to relax the body
5) get 7-8 hours of sleep each night
6) get 15-20 minutes of sunlight daily without sunglasses or sunscreen (use sunscreen and sunglasses after this amount).

7) do something you enjoy to relax, do some of the top 5 things you enjoy in life—especially if you haven't done them in a while
8) express your feelings—don't bottle them up inside, or judge your feelings
9) feel free to cry when you need to, this is a natural expression
10) get support from others—friends, family, groups associations
11) have a "hardy personality" by using these techniques to withstand high amounts of stress
12) get into your own personal "C-Zone" where you balance challenge with mastery and stay just above the "comfort zone."

The Audio CD of this eBook is available at:
www.Nutripoints.com and www.TheMojoCoach.com.

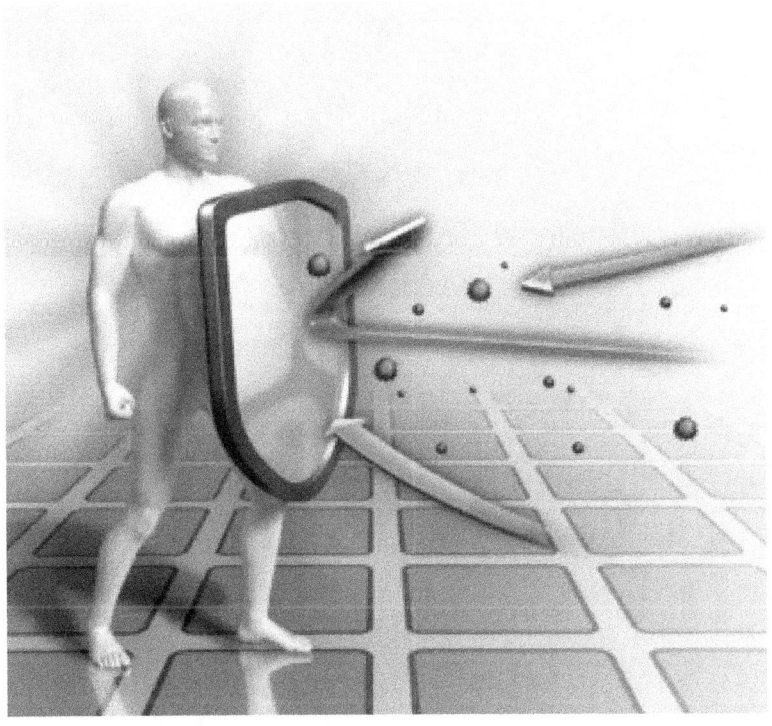

Personal Stress Analysis

List 3 reasons we are having more stress than ever today:

1._____

_____

2._____

_____

3._____

_____

What are some of your body's physical reactions to stress:

_____

_____

_____

_____

_____

_____

What are some of your personal long-term symptoms of stress?

_____

_____

_____

_____

_____

_____

_____

What are some of the stress-related diseases you are at risk for if symptoms go on too long?

_____

_____

_____

_____

_____

_____

List the top 5 most stressful things right now in your life:

1._____

_____

2._____

_____

3._____

_____

4._____

_____

5._____

_____

List 3 things you can do to decrease or eliminate some of these stressors in your life:

1._____

_____

_____

_____

2._____

_____

_____

_____

3._____

_____

_____

_____

Which stressors in your life are things you can't change or do anything about that you can change your perception of to enable you to "let go" and possibly turn a negative into a positive?

_____

_____

_____

_____

_____

_____

_____

Which coping mechanisms are you using, and which can you add to your life to help you burn off the effects of inevitable stress?

Using:_____

_____

_____

_____

_____

_____

_____

Will add and use:_____

_____

_____

_____

_____

_____

_____

_____

Where do you fall in the scheme of riding your own personal stress wave? In the Drone Zone of boredom? In the Panic Zone of stressed out? Or in the "C" Zone going between challenge and mastery? If you are not in the "C" Zone, what do you need to do to get and stay there?

My Zone:_____

_____

_____

_____

_____

_____

3-Day Hydration Log
Goal—Eight 8 oz. Glasses Water/Day

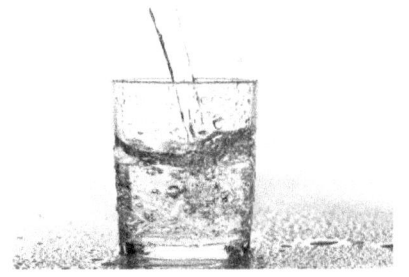

Day One

Drink   **Amount**

_____

_____

_____

_____

_____

_____

_____

Day Two

Drink   **Amount**

_____

_____

_____

_____

_____

_____

_____

_____

Day Three

Drink   **Amount**

_____

_____

_____

_____

_____

_____

_____

7-Day Sleep Tracker
Goal—7 to 8 Hours/Night

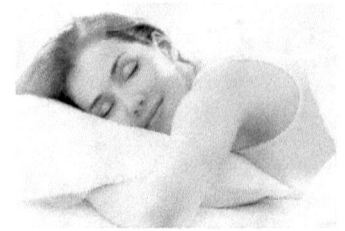

Date   **Hours of Sleep**

_____

_____

_____

_____

_____

_____

3-Day Stress Diary

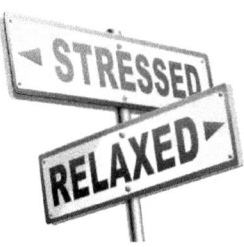

Day One

Stress Score (0-10, 10 highest):_____

Event:_____

_____

_____

Reaction/Response:_____

_____

_____

_____

What I Could Have Done Better:_____

_____

_____

Day Two

Stress Score (0-10, 10 highest):_____

Event:_____

_____

_____

_____

Reaction/Response:_____

_____

_____

_____

What I Could Have Done Better:_____

_____

_____

Day Three

Stress Score (0-10, 10 highest):_____

Event:_____

_____

_____

_____

Reaction/Response:_____

_____

_____

_____

What I Could Have Done Better:_____

_____

_____

Notes and Thoughts

Notes and Thoughts

Notes and Thoughts

Notes and Thoughts

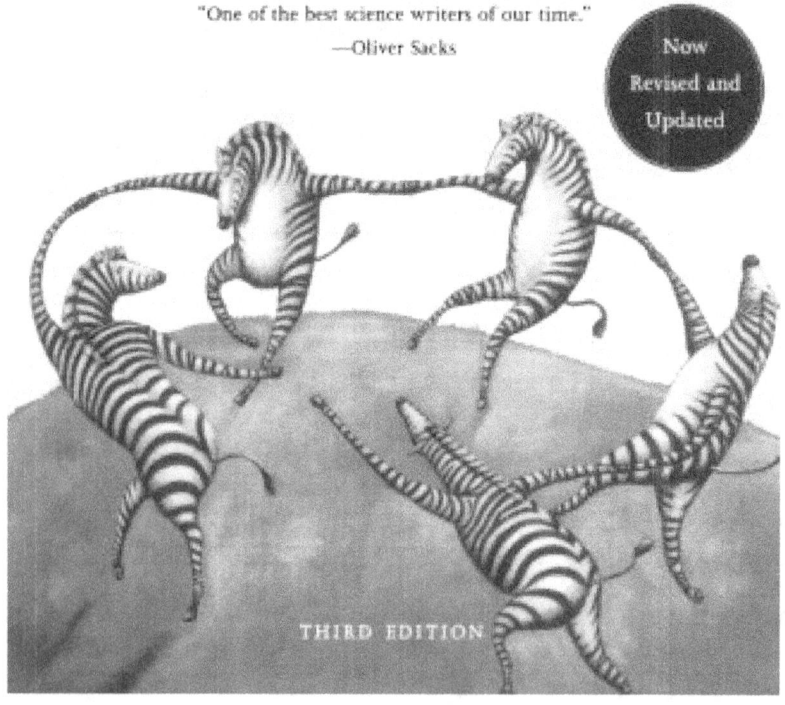

ROBERT M. SAPOLSKY
Author of *A Primate's Memoir*

WHY ZEBRAS DON'T GET ULCERS

The Acclaimed Guide to Stress,
Stress-Related Diseases, and Coping

"One of the best science writers of our time."
—Oliver Sacks

Now
Revised and
Updated

THIRD EDITION

IS IT WORTH DYING FOR?

How to Make Stress Work for You— Not Against You

"I have the utmost admiration for Dr. Eliot's book,
as I have for the man himself."
—Norman Cousins, author of *Anatomy of an Illness*

by Dr. Robert S. Eliot and Dennis L. Breo

Introduction by Michael E. DeBakey, M.D.

IS TYPE A BEHAVIOR KILLING YOU—
BUT YOU'RE TOO AMBITIOUS TO BE TYPE B?
ENTER...

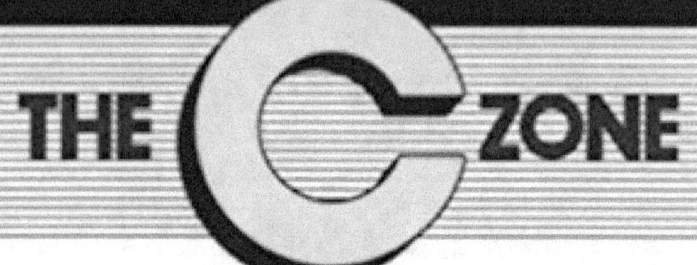

THE C ZONE

PEAK
PERFORMANCE
UNDER
PRESSURE

Robert Kriegel, Ph.D., and
Marilyn Harris Kriegel, Ph.D.

"A winner of a book, and badly needed."
Thomas J. Peters, co-author,
IN SEARCH OF EXCELLENCE

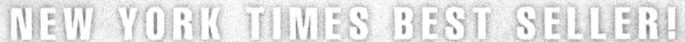

The **BREAKTHROUGH** method that allows you to
easily choose healthy foods you love!

Nutripoints

HEALTHY EATING — MADE SIMPLE!

75 pts SPINACH

100's of
NEW FOODS
& DRINKS!
3600+ Foods
Rated!

30 pts TOMATOES

Choose
Foods
That Count
the Most

12.5 pts RASPBERRIES

Stop
Calculating
Carbs &
Protein

1 pt PRETZELS

-5 pts JELLY BEANS

Dr. Roy Vartabedian & KATHY MATTHEWS
FOREWORD BY KENNETH H. COOPER, M.D.

Juice Plus+® Top-Rated Nutritionals
Rated A+ by Nutripoints

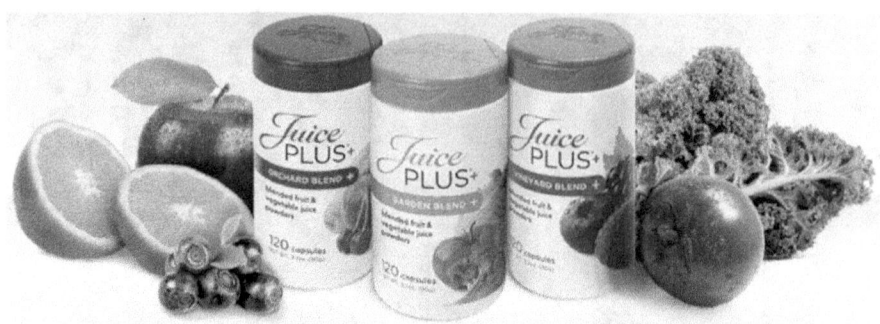

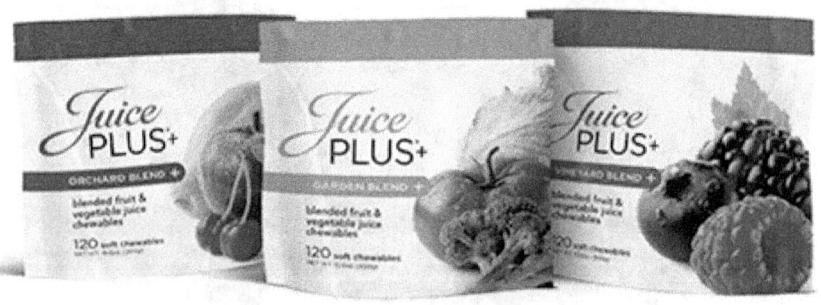

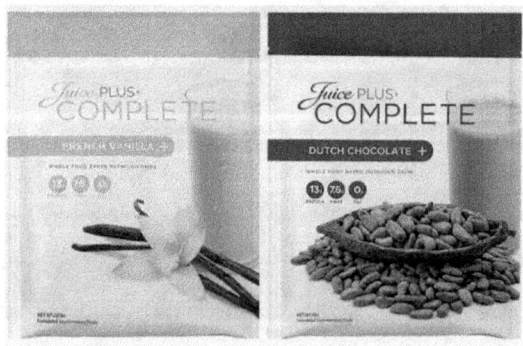

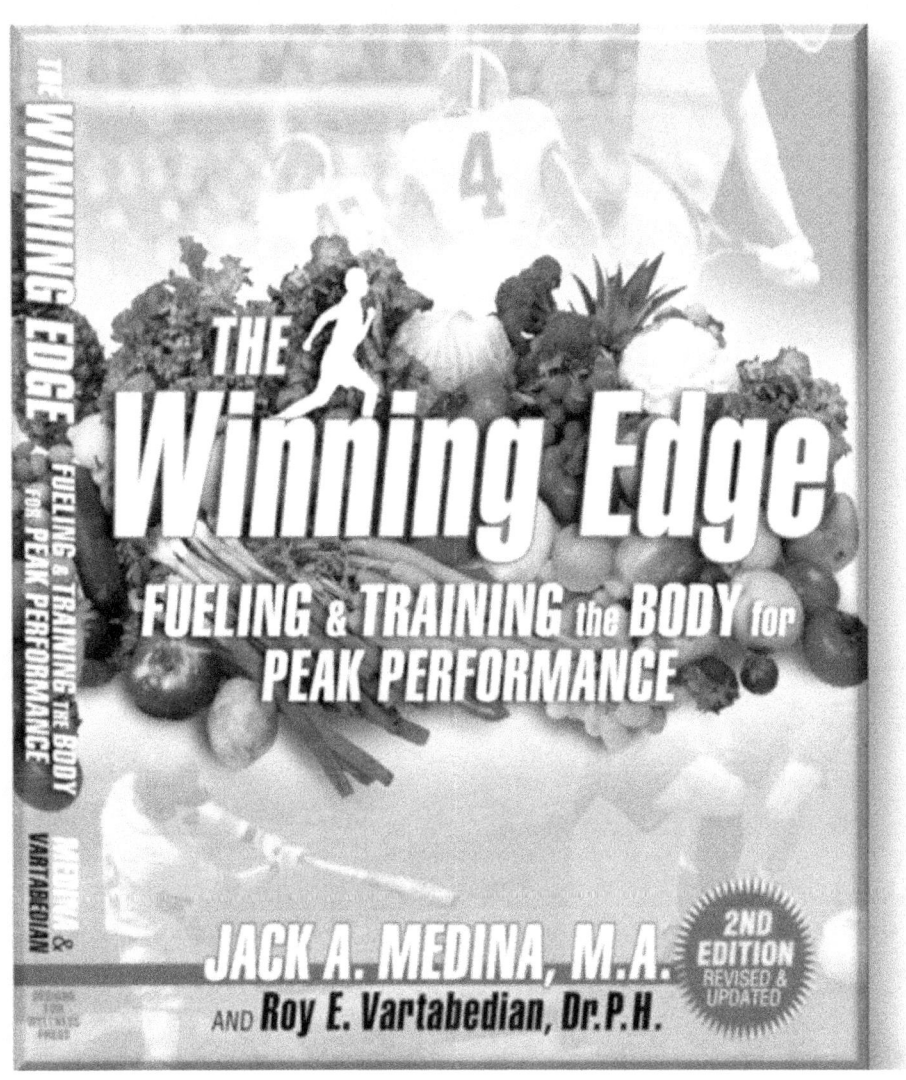

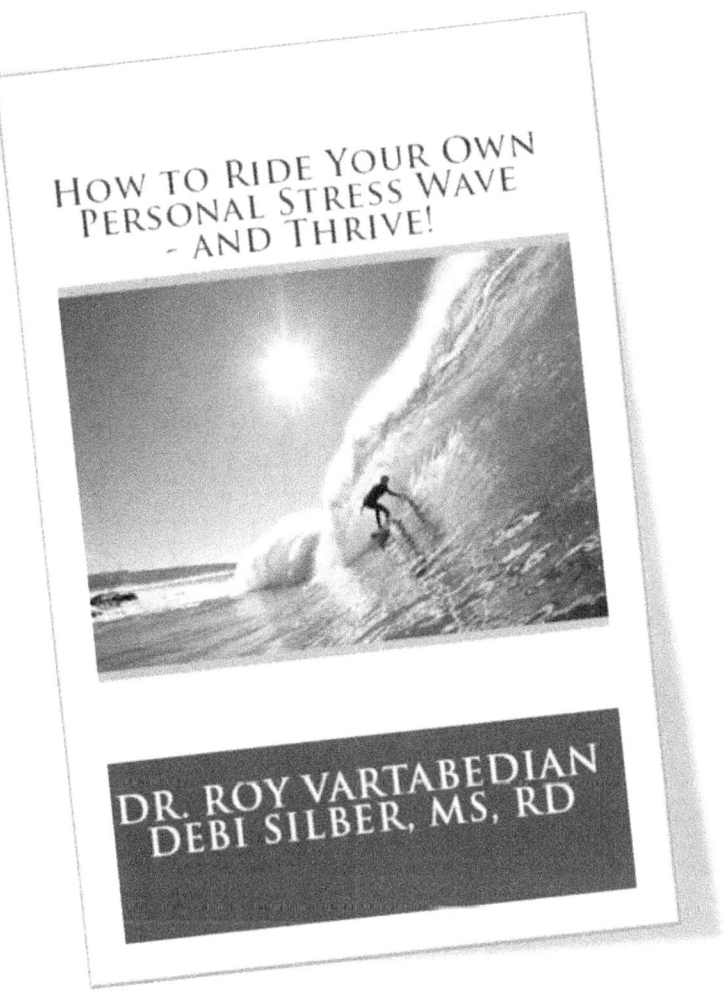

How to Ride Your Own Personal Stress Wave - and Thrive!

DR. ROY VARTABEDIAN
DEBI SILBER, MS, RD

To order additional copies of this book
and for large volume discounts go to:

www.Nutripoints.com

or call (760) 458-4993.

www.ingramcontent.com/pod-product-compliance
Lightning Source LLC
Chambersburg PA
CBHW071222280526
45787CB00002B/770